GLYCEMIC DIET

FOR HEALTH

Glycemic Diet For Health

Using The Glycemic Index Diet Plan To
Lose Weight Fast And Live A Healthy Life

Andy Jackson

TABLE OF CONTENT

Chapter 1: Glycemic Index

This book would show you how Glycemic Index is calculated and used more effectively as a guide to healthier living. This guide would show that using the Glycemic Index could be done easily and the tremendous benefits that follow. From this book, you will discover how controlling your food intake based on the Glycemic index allows you to reduce the risk of diabetes, lose weight and lower your cholesterol levels.

Glycemic Index is directly linked to the sugars in your food and how they are absorbed over time. This index measures carbohydrates, which are made of both simple and complex molecules. The Glycemic index ranks the effects of having this food on your system.

By understanding these effects and following certain simple guidelines, you would be able to recognize the food by the Glycemic index and take better food. From here, you would discover that many carbohydrates are actually very helpful to you and you don't have to avoid all the carbohydrates as many diets recommend.

This book goes into depth about how high and low blood sugar levels affect your well-being. You would understand this link between the Glycemic index and controlling diabetes. You could even substantially reduce the risk of becoming diabetic.

As you read this book and become more similar with what this Glycemic Index is all about, you would know the different benefits of it. From here, you would find that making the best choices would come naturally with little effort required.

Chapter 2: What Is The Glycemic Index

Simply put, the Glycemic Index is a type of rating system for food where any form of carbohydrate has a certain numerical value assigned to it. This is based on its components and how the food affects our body's sugar levels.

A Canadian professor, Dr. David Jenkins, developed this concept of rating index. He felt that a better system was required because of the popularity of certain diets like South Beach and Atkins which was against the use of all carbohydrates and many form of fats.

He wanted to prove that it was not accurate to categorize carbohydrates as simple and complex. Most carbohydrates are simply too complex to label them in such a manner. He wanted to prove to the world that any foods we eat affect our bodies' blood sugar levels in a different way. Generally speaking, when food breaks down in your digestive system, the food components are absorbed into our blood stream and affect our system immediately.

Food that break down instantly and have a high glucose or sugar levels would give us a quick spiked feeling of euphoria. This is commonly referred to as 'sugar high'.

Some other foods break down slower and release their starches, nutrients and sugars over a longer period of time. This avoids the rapid increases to our sugar levels and ensures that our insulin levels are low.

In this book, we would explain what glucose and insulin are and how they would affect our bodies and health. Dr. Jenkins proved that many carbohydrates are very healthy and shouldn't be avoided just because they are carbohydrates.

From his research, he also encountered some surprising results on the food that he tested. Many of the foods that are considered 'diet food' were very high on the Glycemic Index.

Until now, Dr. Jenkins has been working in this field of dietary science. He is continually pursuing this link between diet and health. He has proved the theory that taking a certain diet would improve of eliminate certain health issues like diabetes, cancer or a lot of other severe diseases.

Chapter 3: How Is Glycemic Index In Foods Determined

The Glycemic Index uses pure glucose as the control food and rates other food based on it. The standard of control, glucose or white bread, is given a rating of 100 and other foods are tested to evaluate how they would affect a person's blood sugar levels, lipid levels and insulin levels. Every food you take would be given a rating number and given either of these category - *High, Medium or Low* - on the Glycemic Index.

A food is considered in the High Glycemic Index if they have a rating of 70 and above. A rating of 56-69 would be considered Medium; while a rating of below 55 would be considered Low. The testing of a Glycemic Index is very scientific and takes into consideration the test subjects who undergo these multiple tests with the same food and with the control food, which is the glucose.

The test subject would first fast for a minimum of 12 hours. Then, he would have his blood drawn and tested. From there, he would be given a specified amount of glucose, which in most cases, is around 50 grams.

Then, their blood would be drawn and their blood sugar levels tested at different times throughout the testing period. This is to determine the control level in the individual. In most circumstances, this exact glucose test is done a few times in the same test subject to have a more accurate result.

Once all the blood sugar levels have been determined, they are plotted on a graph which shows the curve of how high the sugar levels rose and how long they would remain elevated. From here, the next step is to take the same individual on another day, after a 12 hour period and ask them to eat a food sample that is tested.

Simply put, the amount in grams of carbohydrates in the test food must equal the grams of carbohydrates in the glucose control test. Depending on the tested item, the quantity of food that the test subject needs to eat may be very little in foods that are dense in carbohydrates. In other circumstances, the test subject would need to eat an enormous amount of food that has little carbohydrates to reach 50 grams of carbohydrates.

As an example, if the test subject need to ingest pure glucose of 50 grams of carbohydrates and the tested food is banana, the test subject would need to take an equivalent of 50 grams of carbohydrates in banana.

From here, their blood would be drawn and tested. This is done at the same time with the control test with the glucose. The blood sugar levels results would be entered to the same graph as the glucose tests. The results would then be compared. These 'banana' tests are repeated over the next few days with the same test subject to ensure more reliable results.

Then, this testing process with the banana is repeated with different test subjects.

This is the sort of testing that is done on every food that has a certain type of sugar or carbohydrates in it. There are numerous tests being done to determine the Glycemic Index of every food.

After all these 'banana tests', the glucose control tests and specified food tests have been completed; the results are determined. The number for the glucose test is set to 100 and the food that is being tested is graphed and measured up to determine its affects to the person's blood sugar levels, in relation to glucose.

It was found from tests that banana affects a person's blood sugar levels only 53% as much compared to the levels that pure glucose would affect them. Therefore, a banana is rated as 53 on the Glycemic Index. This puts it in the Medium Glycemic Index range.

Does this mean that bananas are good or bad for you?

We would better understand the Glycemic Index results and how to incorporate them into your daily diet later in this book. In the next chapter, we would look at the common myth that all carbohydrates are bad and should be avoided at all cost.

Chapter 4: Good Carbs

When medical practitioners start looking as to what makes the average diet and why most people tend to gain weight, they first looked at the food pyramid.

Carbohydrate has slowly become a word associated with a bad diet practice. It advances the notion that any food with carbohydrates (or sugar) shouldn't be consumed. Some people even treat carbohydrates like poison and can't bear the sight of it. It is almost a religious practice for some people to eliminate carbohydrates from their diet.

Upon this new fad of "low carb", the food industries started to take a turn. Never one to miss a money-making opportunity, they come out with packaged food or restaurant food selling this "low carb" concept. This idea has made them a tremendous amount of money.

However, this sort of thinking is too simplistic and not all carbohydrates are bad. This is proven by the developers of this Glycemic Index. Researchers of this index wanted to see qualitative scientific evidence that prove that all carbohydrates were unhealthy. Their findings prove otherwise.

They discovered that different types of carbohydrates affect blood sugar levels and insulin release to varying degrees. They were surprised to also discover that many so-called 'bad carbohydrates' weren't bad while others that seem healthy actually spiked blood levels tremendously. A good example of such food is watermelon. The Glycemic Index of watermelon is 70, in the high range. It is commonly considered healthy, but this index proved otherwise.

Although watermelon have very few calories, it has very high content of natural sugar and easily spikes your blood sugar levels This forces the body to release insulin to counteract and lower these levels. In the later chapter, we would learn more about the consequences to insulin is continuously released to keep blood sugar level.

On the other hand, certain food which are artificially sweetened or peanuts have a score of below 30. This makes them better choices when following a Glycemic Index diet. They wouldn't spike your blood sugar levels and would provide a slow energy release instead over a period of time. This sort of food provides you with more energy and you would feel full for a longer period.

Chapter 5: Effects Of Glucose

At its purest form, glucose is a form of simple sugar found in many of the food we eat. The body uses glucose to produce energy for its functioning. It is a molecule which is made up of several cells that could be extracted from starchy grains. This includes wheat, corn, rice and potatoes. The moment the glucose is extracted from these plants, it is added into any number of food processes to enhance and sweeten the flavor.

The most common food additive in the United States is derived from cornstarch. It is heated in a water solution for a couple of hours at relatively low temperature and this result in breaking down the starch into even smaller particles.

A common species of fungus would then be added and this promotes the starch to break down to the basic element of glucose. The mixture is purified and concentrated until the glucose is in crystal form.

The crystals are then packages into cubes and sold to food industries. Besides this, there are also other forms of sugar that are used in food packaging such as fructose which is derived from fruits, vegetables and honey.

Generally speaking, fructose is sweeter than glucose. For those who have diabetes, fructose is recommended. However, it has to be noted that while every cell in the human body could metabolize glucose, only the liver can process fructose. All forms of sugar would raise blood sugar levels and create an insulin resistance.

While the body ingests glucose or other sort of carbohydrates, it would break it down to its simplest form and use them for energy. Most of this energy in your body is produced from carbohydrates. Sugar molecules are broken down and converted into carbon dioxide and oxygen molecules and this keeps the body functioning. This conversion translates into our metabolism - the way our body efficiently turn foods into energy.

Besides that, glucose is also the primary sources of energy to ensure proper functioning of organs and brain. This would explain why you feel a feeling of euphoria after you ingest a food item which is high in glucose.

A great number of people would feel dizzy and lightheaded when their blood sugar levels become too high or low. The human body regulates itself on an even keel and when it is overfed or underfed with sugar, it would try to overcompensate. As such, the body would release insulin to compensate for these actions.

You would feel certain symptoms. This includes an immediate reaction from having too much glucose. After that, you would suffer from the counteractions your body has to perform to react to our actions. It's like a vicious cycle. Therefore, it is very important to know how our bodies work, what insulin is and its purpose. In the next chapter, we would learn more about insulin. From there, you would realize how valuable but fragile insulin is.

Chapter 6: About Insulin

Insulin is a certain hormone produced and released from the pancreas. The main purpose of insulin is to let the body's cell know that they are fed sufficiently and would need no further nutrients. The insulin resupplies and routes the extra glucose from the food you eat into the liver and muscles to be stored as a kind of short term 'fat' which is used first before other fat deposits when energy is needed again.

Simply put, each time you feed your body too much with fats, sugars, proteins; your body would store these extras and burn them instead of the extra weight and fat already deposited in your body.

When you eat a lot of high Glycemic Index food on a consistent basis, it would force your insulin to be released continuously. "Insulin resistance" happens when you ask your insulin to react to this great dosage of glucose and insulin couldn't keep up with the workload and diminishes.

Those people who have no insulin response or if they have low insulin levels are considered diabetic. These people's bodies can't digest and route the glucose, any sugar or carbohydrates. As such, they would need to provide their biology with an artificial atmosphere by having an insulin injection every day.

There are tremendous complications when one has diabetes. It would be covered in depth later in this book. If you aren't familiar with diabetes, take some time to research it even after you have read this book. It is very common to think it isn't serious. However, diabetes is a very serious condition that leads to many complications and in more severe situations, death.

Therein lies the power of following the recommendations of the Glycemic Index. As you lead more about Glycemic Loading and to incorporate the Insulin Index, you would avoid the risk of developing diabetes. In the next chapter, you would go into greater depth about how to avoid diabetes.

Chapter 7: The Glycemic Index And Diabetes Connection

Once it is clear that is isn't only cookies, candy desserts and cakes which contain sugars and raise our blood sugar, we are in better positioned to reduce our chances of diabetes. Any form of food considered as carbohydrate consists of sugars and starches.

There are certain foods that are not considered "sweet" by your standards, but are full of dextrose, glucose or sucrose. Certain food like pretzels, beets and baked potatoes can raise your blood sugar levels and this forces your body to increase the insulin levels.

When your insulin is over-worked and stop responding to high blood sugar levels, it would show certain symptoms of diabetes. They include being very thirsty a lot of the time and drinking a lot of fluids. Once the insulin levels aren't there anymore, people would complain of a blurred vision, open sores and leg cramps.

Simply put, there are two types of diabetes. It is called Type 1 and Type 2. Type 1 is the more serious of the two and people with Type 1 would have no insulin response to counteract their sugar levels.

Your body can't survive for too long without insulin as it is difficult to avoid certain foods which raise our blood sugar. The body's main sources of energy lie in sugar and starch, which is found in almost every food. Insulin is required to direct the cells and inform them as to how to deal with the fuel that comes in. Without it, the body would malfunction and couldn't handle the energy that comes in.

Those people who are diagnosed with Type 1 diabetes should be supplied with artificial insulin daily through injections. They should also be aware of their daily diet and need to monitor their blood sugar levels throughout the day. This is a lot of hassle.

Although Type 2 diabetes isn't as serious as Type 1, is shouldn't be ignored. It is also very serious, although less severe than Type 1. In Type 2 diabetes, the patient would have certain levels of insulin but find that it doesn't do the required job effectively.

Those who have Type 2 diabetes can control their situation with the right diet, regular exercise and medication. They also need to regularly monitor their sugar levels. However, many people don't take their condition seriously and this only worsens their situation.

The excessive eating of High Glycemic and High Insulin Index food is the major cause which leads to the failure of insulin response. It is very important that you don't overwork the body in such a manner.

If you aren't diabetic, it is unimportant or not recommended to avoid all carbohydrates and sweets. However, you need to be moderate anything you eat. Limit yourself to the food categorized as Low Glycemic Index. Eat lesser of food which are of Medium Glycemic Index and even lesser of food which are of High Glycemic Index.

The moment the damage is done and you are diagnosed with diabetes, it is probably too late to reverse this condition with the right diet. Diabetes is a very chronic condition and once your body stops producing insulin, it doesn't heal itself. Therefore, always look to eat healthy now before diabetes strikes into your life.

Among the complication that comes with diabetes include hypoglycemia. This is a condition where there is insufficient supply of glucose which creates neurological problems. Other complications include heart disease, blindness, impotence and nerve damage.

From here, it is clear that those people who suffer from diabetes need to treat their condition properly as it results in more serious complications in the future. You need to keep diabetes under control and following the Glycemic Index is the way to lower the risk of developing diabetes. This would be shared in the later chapters of this book.

Chapter 8: Incorporating The Insulin Index

The Insulin Index is similar to the Glycemic Index. The only difference is that during the testing, insulin levels in the blood are tested instead of blood sugar or glucose levels.

The results are similar and the differences are that when you are testing the food for raised insulin levels, those proteins and lean meats were found to raise your insulin levels as well. Just by following certain guidelines, you can easily incorporate the Insulin Index with the Glycemic Index.

Simply put, foods that are rich in protein could mimic a sugar response in your body once they break down. This may include beef, lamb, eggs, shellfish and hard cheese. Because they are rich in protein, vitamins and minerals; you can't avoid them completely. However, a person's diet shouldn't be made up solely based on these choices and on an irregular basis.

As like for any advice, you should always do anything in moderation. Even the best food in the world wouldn't be good if you take it excessively. The body needs different nutrients and the only way to do this is to eat anything and don't just focus on eating one.

Our bodies are tremendous systems where would try to adapt to any conditions you put it under. If we starve it, it would still be able to hold on to the last pound of fat to survive. However, in this process, other bodily functions would suffer.

We may not be able to see the damage we cause to our systems in our overindulgence of certain food but it doesn't mean that we are not causing our body harm.

Binge eating may not immediately result in diseases or serious conditions. However, we need to realize that small things build up and create problems. Many conditions like weight gain, headaches, insomnia and moodiness can be traced to our eating habits.

Glycemic Index and Insulin Index are used to achieve the same goal - which is to inform people of the reaction and hard work we put our bodies under when we take certain food.

When we make poor choices, we eventually force our bodies to work extremely hard until our systems fail.

The body is like a complicated machine. If we overwork them and never do any maintenance, it would break down over time. We may not even notice the changes when our insulin levels are high but your liver, pancreas, heart and brain would feel the strain and make these adjustments to your eating habits and lifestyle choices. Regardless, even the strongest body can't handle the pressure over time.

Our insulin levels wouldn't be able to counter the high blood sugars in our system and creates problems for our body. This includes heart disease, heart failure, diabetes and rapid weight gain. On the other hand, if you follow the recommendation of eating food from the low ranges of the Insulin and Glycemic range, you can notice improvements in your health gradually.

So, this is the power of incorporating the Insulin and Glycemic Index. You would improve your overall health and would also reduce the risk of certain diseases.

Chapter 9: Weight Loss Benefits

Probably the most obvious benefit of the Glycemic Index diet is weight loss over a period of time. We all definitely want a healthier heart and lower cholesterol, but we also want to lose weight.

In fact, in many people I know of, losing weight is perhaps even more important that being healthy. The great side benefits of weight loss through following the Glycemic Index recommendation is perhaps worth it.

This Glycemic Index was developed to control blood sugar from dips and spikes. This would allow a more constant insulin levels. Without a doubt, the food choices we make following the Glycemic Index are food that allow a more natural weight loss and help us maintain this weight.

This food which keep our sugar and insulin levels on a healthy basis are the similar foods which gives us a longer and more constant feeling of fullness. When our energy levels are fed continuously, we don't have to keep on eating.

Without a doubt, everyone has had this feeling of euphoria after eating food which is high in sugars and carbohydrates. However, this 'high' comes with an equal 'low'. This happens every time we put our body through this kind of situation even if we don't recognize it.

Many people are continuously confused as to why they are hungry very soon after finishing a meal that is made up of High Glycemic Index food. However, it's not because we are hungry but it's just because our hormone have gone through a roller coaster ride and have trouble adjusting to it.

Similarly to a pendulum which swings back and forth, your body reacts to an extreme by correcting it. This swings the pendulum back into the other direction. This extreme back and forth would destroy our health and keep us from losing weight.

Along with any permanent changes you want to make, you need to prepare for it mentally. We may know it logically that what we are doing is harmful to our body but it may become such a bad habit that we become totally helpless in breaking this cycle. We may hate it when our blood sugar levels are low and causes a feeling of depression.

It takes some time and hard work to adjust to this diet but once you focus, this would be much easier. You would learn to focus your joys on other things rather than food and how it makes you feel. From here, following the Glycemic Index would be easy.

Chapter 10: Reduced Diabetes Risk

In the past few chapters, I have shared how the Glycemic Index would affect diabetes. However, there is more to that. The past few chapters were about the potential risks that arise when we overwork our hormone insulin as well as the possible complications that could arise when choosing food that demands a lot from our glucose and insulin levels.

By following the Glycemic index however, you could eliminate the risk of contracting diabetes. When you follow this index, it protects your insulin response from being overtaxed and this keeps your heart, brain and other organs healthier over time.

As a matter of fact, if your diet is solely based on food on the Low Glycemic Index, it would make your insulin more sensitive and responsive. This is a good thing as having insulin which reacts quickly and efficiently to whatever you eat would result in a much healthier individual.

Treat it like a workout for your insulin. When you eat right and make the right choices, you would have your internal systems and organs working well. As such, you would also look healthier.

An even better practice is to add exercise into your daily activity. Even light exercises of around 20 minutes a day could increase the chances of you fighting diabetes. Additionally, you can also avoid other form of diseases, not just diabetes.

You wouldn't want to take your chances with diabetes as it is a very complicated condition. It can be kept in check with a strict diet and medication but it is certainly not a condition you want to contract.

By practicing the recommendations of the Glycemic Index, it would better protect you from developing diabetes. If your family has a history of relatives who have suffered or is suffering from diabetes, then this is really important. You could see what diabetes does to the people you love and wouldn't want to be part of this club.

Therefore, start making better choice today. You don't have to start big. Just start slowly and make small changes every week until a year from now, you can look back and see a completely different person not just from the outside, but from the inside as well.

Chapter 11: Improved Heart Health

It may be difficult to find a direct link between eating foods which are high in starches, sugars and heart disease; but there is definitely a link. When you eat too much of High Glycemic Index food, your system would go into high alert to bring your system back down to a more normal function.

As sugars and starches are the body's main energy source, during the ingestion, our bodies would either try to use it all or store the excess as a quick source of needed fuel. When we overtake foods which are considered in the High Glycemic Index, we ask our body to work harder and the body would slowly feel the burden that we have given it.

Slowly, our blood pressure would increase to ensure that the sugar and insulin in the bloodstream can move as fast as it can. Our heart would also go into a 'marathon mode' to ensure that the blood is moving and increase the oxygen to perform all these tough functions.

This is even more difficult for those people who aren't healthy - those overweight and continuously feed their body with unhealthy food. It isn't hard to see how their heart would wear out our time.

Those who continued with a High Glycemic Index diet were twice more likely to develop a heart attack or heart disease within the next ten years compared to those who follow a Low

Glycemic Index diet. If you are women, you should even treat this more seriously. Over the past few years, women have surpassed men in terms of the number of heart attacks deaths and heart diseases. Generally, women would die within five years of suffering a heart attack.

As this is clear, you can't take this situation lightly. The way for improving this situation is simply by using this Glycemic Index method. This would improve your heart health significantly and should be a major priority in your life.

This is especially so if you have someone in your family history who suffers from heart attacks or strokes. Again, if you focus on Low Glycemic Index food, your heart would be healthier and increases your lifespan.

Chapter 12: Lower Cholesterol

Low Glycemic Index foods are generally those foods which are high in fiber and lower in calories. They are exactly the right kind of foods to eat to ensure that you have a healthy heart and low cholesterol.

Cholesterol is a trace molecule which is found in food which travels in our bloodstream and helps in many important tasks. One of its main functions is to help reform the cell membranes. Besides that, cholesterol also helps in the creation of certain steroid hormones that the body uses.

If our cholesterol aren't ingested, our bodies would suffer. However, there is a big difference between 'good' and 'bad' cholesterol. Bad cholesterol is known as LDL while good cholesterol is known as HDL.

They are very similar in make-up but they are very different in terms of how it affects the body. If you have a high level of HDL in your body, it would help lower your overall cholesterol levels.

This would also keep our arteries clear and ensure our heart is running smoothly. However, if you have high levels of LDL; it means that you have harmful cholesterol. It clogs the arteries and causes heart problems.

It should be reminded that the main supplier of cholesterol to our body is the food we eat. We ourselves have the power to affect the quantity of good or bad cholesterol in our body.

By following the recommendations of the Glycemic Index, you would be able to choose the right foods which helps you lower your cholesterol levels. This would also eliminate other health issues which come with it. One of the main health issues that people may suffer from when they have high cholesterol levels are gallstones.

When you have an excess of cholesterol, your liver would try to process as much as it can. The excess would be absorbed into other organs of the body. Once inside the organs like the gallbladder, the cholesterol would sit and harden. It would develop into very painful gallstones and may need to be surgically removed.

The accepted cholesterol levels are at a ratio of 5:1. This means that for every particle of bad cholesterol (LDL), we should have at least 5 particles of good cholesterol (HDL).

By using the Glycemic Index, you will realize the goal of increasing your good cholesterol while decreasing the bad. You can achieve this goal because the food you eat would help keep your systems running smoothly without spikes. Again, Glycemic Index is valuable in achieving lower cholesterol.

Chapter 13: Glycemic Loading

In chapter 3, I shared about how to rate a banana on a Glycemic Index scale. It was 53, placing it in the medium scale. However, what if you take two bananas instead? Does it mean that the Glycemic Index is double? No, Glycemic Index is always constant.

However, you have doubled the carbohydrate and sugar amount that your body needs to process. If you ate a banana now, rest for a few hours and then eat another, your system wouldn't need to work as hard. It may seem a bit confusing at the beginning but it is just pure common sense.

The Glycemic Loading is to take the Glycemic Index a little further. This formula takes into account the relationship between the Glycemic Index and the carbohydrate amount in each food that you take.

During the testing of all the food on the Glycemic Index, the measurement used was always 50 grams. In many cases, 50 grams of a food is a lot. This is considerably more than most people would eat in a serving.

However, it is still important to ensure the test results are consistent. Simply put, the control food for all the Glycemic Index testing for 50 grams of glucose, which is simply carbohydrates. This means that every item of tested food is compared to an equal 50 grams worth of carbohydrates.

It doesn't mean that they weigh carrots until it was 50 grams in weight. It meant that they need to eat enough carrots until they have consumed 50 grams of carbohydrates in the carrots consumed.

That is a hell lot of carrots. In simpler terms, half a cup of cooked carrots has 8 grams of carbohydrates. Therefore, each test subject needs to eat more than 3 cups of cooked carrots in order to measure up to 50 grams of carbohydrates.

The difference of Glycemic Load is that it would take the information from the Glycemic Index and calculate to reflect a more sensible serving size. As such, the rating would be reduced and many items which are on the High Glycemic Index would make more sense.

Glycemic Load gives a more practical overview of the food on the Glycemic Index. This allows you to apply the practical information into your diet. In the later chapter, I would share an easy formula and how you can count the Glycemic Load for the food you eat.

Chapter 14: Recognize Low Glycemic Index Foods

Many of the foods which are Low Glycemic Index may be familiar to you. You would need to shed some old ideas about the kinds of foods which you perceive as nothing but 'diet' foods.

The foods considered as Low Glycemic Index are foods which are healthy and keeps your blood sugar level low. They are great for ensuring your body runs smoothly. Besides that, some of the foods are extremely delicious. You wouldn't have to suffer according to the old belief that dieting means eating foods which are horrible in taste.

Simply put, foods which are Low Glycemic are food which is comprised of an abundance of fiber or whole grains. This would include pasta, breads, rice, yogurt and any variety of beans or lentils. This also includes fresh fruits and vegetables.

Before you even know, you would be able to look at a food and know if it is a kind of food which would help you lose weight and reduce the chances of you developing diabetes.

It would also lower your cholesterol and promote a healthier heart. The moment you are more familiar with Low Glycemic Index food, you would be astonished that you won't be attracted by any other type of unhealthy food.

Chapter 15: How To Calculate Glycemic Load

As shared in chapter 13, Glycemic Load is a method of ranking any food that you eat to determine more information of what the Glycemic Index shows. This involves a certain calculation to determine the Glycemic Load.

The Glycemic Load calculation is a simple multiplication. You multiply the food's Glycemic Index rating with the amount of grams of carbohydrates in uses in the serving size you eat.

If the Glycemic Index rating of a food is below 100, use a decimal point so that you know it is less than one. For example, potato has a high Glycemic Index rating of 85 while the number of grams of carbohydrates is 37. Simply multiple 0.85 with 37 and you would get 31.45. Therefore, potato has a Glycemic Load of 31. This makes a good choice in your daily diet.

This shows that Glycemic Index is still very useful in providing information and how Glycemic Load takes the information and makes it more practical for us to use on a daily basis. Generally, the average Glycemic Load range is lower than the Glycemic Index. If the Glycemic Load of a food is above 50, it is considered high.

Many nutritionists recommend keeping the total number of your daily Glycemic Load to be fewer than 150. This makes it much easier than counting calories or fat grams. As such, it makes it easier to make better choices.

This information of how many grams of carbohydrates in your food can be found by simply looking at the nutritional label on the packaging. Simply find the number listed there and multiple with the Glycemic Index rating. This is a great tool for enhancing weight loss and improving your general health.

Chapter 16: Glycemic Index Of Common Foods

In this chapter, is the Glycemic Index for common food which is a valuable guide for helping you make diet choices every day. To start, we would look at those foods which are commonly considered as High on the Glycemic Index.

You should limit and eat these foods only occasionally. When one were to look at this list, one would be shocked to find that certain food like rice cakes, watermelon or baked potatoes are in it. They seem like healthy choices, but not according to the Glycemic Index.

In order for the testing to be done, it had to be consistent and scientific. The food need to be tested in equal amounts of carbohydrates, which means that watermelon had to consumed in massive quantities in order for the test to be equal. However, watermelon has a lot of natural sweetness and sugar but has low amount of carbohydrates. As such watermelon need to be eaten in very large quantities and these substantially the blood sugar level.

This is where Glycemic Load value becomes important. By using the Glycemic Index of watermelon, which is 0.72 and multiply it by 5 grams of carbohydrates in a slice of watermelon, you would get the Glycemic Index of 3.6. As such, even though watermelons are known as High Glycemic Index food, it is considered low with the Glycemic Load system.

This is similar to potatoes and rice cakes, although to a lesser extent. They raise blood sugar levels more than brown rice and whole grain pastas.

However, they are loaded with other nutrients and vitamins which make it foolish to avoid it altogether. Use your own good judgment and common sense.

Once you get this concept, it isn't hard or takes a lot of thought. You just need to be aware of how your body functions and what to eat to ensure that it operates better.

In the list below is a list of food and its Glycemic Index rating. Remember to limit the intake as much as you can.

Food which are High Glycemic Index (over 70)

- Baked Potato - 85
- Bagel - 72
- Cheerios -74
- Cream of Wheat - 74
- Doughnut - 76
- French Fries - 76
- Honey -73
- Jelly Beans - 80
- Mashed Potatoes - 73
- Rice Cakes - 82
- Rice Crispies - 82
- Rye Bread - 76
- Watermelon - 72
- White Bread - 70

Now, we will look at the Medium Glycemic Index food. These are food that you should limit but can take more than those with High Glycemic Index.

Choose them more than those in the High Glycemic Index list. If you see anything in the list that seems too good to be true, the best way is to calculate the Glycemic Load value.

This book has already covered how foods are tested and how much of the food may need to be tested to ensure that in order to ensure a level playing field. If you are not sure of the index rating, the best way is to calculate the Glycemic Load to get a more accurate value. Below is a list of the Medium Glycemic Index food.

Food which are Medium Glycemic Index (56-69)

- Angel Food Cake - 67
- Beets - 64
- Blueberry Muffin - 59
- Bran Muffin - 60
- Cheese Pizza - 60
- Couscous - 65
- Hamburger Bun - 61
- Ice Cream - 61
- Mac & Cheese - 64
- Oatmeal - 65
- Orange Juice - 56
- Pea Soup - 66
- Canned Peaches - 58
- Pineapple - 66
- Pita Bread - 57

- Raisins - 64

- Sourdough Bread - 57

- Taco Shells - 69

- Wheat Thins - 67

- White Rice - 56

- Whole Wheat Bread - 69

Next, is the list of food considered as Low Glycemic Index. These are food that you should focus eating. Most healthy diets are made up of these foods.

As with the high and medium ratings, this list would even surprise you. In the list, you would find Snickers Bar and Spaghetti, food that are often considered something you need to avoid.

Again, remember that it took 50 grams of carbohydrates to compare with the control of 50 carbohydrates of glucose. It only needs a small portion of Snickers to equal 50 grams of carbs. This means that only a small portion of the bar is used to perform the tests.

This is the complete differenced with watermelon. While watermelon needs a huge portion to achieve the goal of 50 carbohydrates, Snickers bar only need a small portion.

As such, a more accurate method is to use Glycemic Load again. With the information provided, we can see that Snickers Bar gets a rating of 80. This is considered high and something you should avoid. This is a list of Low Glycemic Index food.

Food which are Low Glycemic Index (under 55)

- Brown Rice - 55
- Apple Juice - 41
- Baked Beans - 48
- Banana - 53
- Broccoli - 6
- Cooked Carrots - 39
- Cauliflower - 6
- Cheese Tortellini - 50
- Fresh Cherries - 22
- Chocolate - 49
- Grapefruit - 25
- Grapes - 43
- Low-fat Ice Cream - 50
- Kidney Beans - 52
- Kiwifruit - 52

- Lentils - 28
- Lettuce - 7
- Linguine - 55
- Macaroni - 45
- Soy Milk - 30
- Oatmeal Cookies - 55
- Fresh Orange Juice - 52
- Fresh Peach - 28
- Peanuts - 14
- Peas - 48
- Popcorn - 55
- Potato Chips - 54
- Pound Cake - 54
- Snickers Bar - 40
- Spaghetti - 41
- Special K Cereal - 54
- Spinach - 12

- Sweet Corn - 55

- Sweet Potato - 54

- Tomato - 15

This isn't a comprehensive list of food because it would take many pages to list all the food there is and the Glycemic Index. However, this gives you a rough idea.

With time, you are able to follow the Glycemic Index effortlessly. You don't have to feel the need to log every single item you eat. You wouldn't need to bring a calculator with you every time you eat. As you familiar yourself with the food that are listed, you would become a master of this.

If you have a food which you aren't sure of its Glycemic Index of Glycemic Load rating, head on to this website: www.glycemicload.com -

which has a great list of thousands of food and its rating. Once you have the Glycemic Index rating, it is very simple to calculate the Glycemic Load. From here you would get an even clearer picture of how healthy your diet is.

In the very next chapter, we would show you show guidelines that you should practice when following the Glycemic Index. These are very helpful advice about what to do and a few practical advices to get the most out of this eating system.

Chapter 17: Guidelines Of The Glycemic Index Diet

❖ Enjoy as much of fresh fruits and vegetables as you can.

❖ Choose whole grains over processed whenever you can. This is clearly written in the packaging of the food.

❖ Don't mix too many foods together. Try eating as many foods as you can alone and make sure it is natural.

❖ If possible, add vinegar or no-fat vinaigrette dressing in the food you eat. This is because vinegar is acidic and lowers the food's Glycemic Index rating.

❖ Make sure that you eat at least one food from the Low Glycemic Index rating at each meal.

❖ See the big picture. Some food may be high or medium on the Glycemic Index but have nutrients that are hard to find in other food.

❖ Don't overeat or take too large a portion. This would make it hard for your digestive system.

❖ Try as many type of food as you can from the Low Glycemic Index list.

❖ Don't forget about eating fats and calories. For example, peanuts are in the Low Glycemic Index but it is not good to eat it often. It would raise your blood sugar but it would pack your body with fats and calories.

❖ Eat foods which are high in fiber. Fiber takes longer to digest. As such, you would feel full longer and maintain your blood sugars at a steadier level for a few hours.

❖ Always take beans. Most beans fall under the Low Glycemic index and are packed with food nutritional value.

❖ Breakfast is the most important meal and you should start it with a Low Glycemic Index breakfast. See if you can choose whole grains, fresh fruits and vegetables. Starting your day such makes it very easy to maintain your blood glucose levels throughout the day.

❖ Eat you meals at a regular time.

❖ Don't eat too much of unhealthy food like caffeine, salt or alcohol. Your body has problem correcting this imbalance.

❖ Don't be discouraged if you find it hard to keep up. Creating a habit is difficult. We would fall in our habits from time to time but the thing you must do is to come back up and continue doing it.

- ❖ Eat a variety of good foods daily.
- ❖ Be aware of the types of fats you choose. Fat is a necessary nutrient. However, not all fat are the same. Try to use fats which are better for your heart like canola and olive oil.
- ❖ Plan your menus beforehand. Look to shop with a list and buy plenty of fresh fruits and vegetables.
- ❖ Look for various Glycemic Index recipes for variety. There is a good link in the resources chapter. It is a book filled with great food recipes. You can check out how you can cook great food from this link: http://gluttenfreerecipes.wellbeingvalley.com/

Chapter 18: Final Notes

Once you are familiar with the guidelines, it would slowly become effortless. From here, you would realize that this doesn't prohibit you from eating the food that you choose but only recommends that you make the best choice in the situation you are in.

In perfect scientific conditions, this Glycemic Index is infallible. However, our lives are not like in laboratory. There are a lot of external factors which would influence the Glycemic Index.

Earlier in this book, I mentioned that eating foods together with other foods would change the Glycemic Index. However, this doesn't mean is a bad thing. It could be a good thing as well. If you choose a higher rated item and eat a low rated food together with it, this would lower the Glycemic Index of the higher rated food.

As a matter of fact, rather than eating a high Glycemic Index food as a meal, it would be better to add a low index food to slow down your digestion. This would help your body deal better with the higher blood sugar.

Besides that, the way your food is being prepared can change the Index. However, Glycemic Index doesn't lose its value because it provides invaluable information. Even if the Glycemic Index is off by a few points, this system still help to let you know which foods are better than the rest. The whole purpose of

Glycemic Index is to ensure that your life is lived more effortlessly while you choose the best food and become healthier every day.

Without a doubt, there would be some of you who need a bit of structure. This is normal as it is very hard to make some of those changes. These changes take a lot of time and it is very hard to change certain lifelong habits.

A common method of ensuring that you can implement this diet better is to purchase a blood glucose meter and test your glucose levels after each meal. These meters are similar to the one that diabetics use to test their blood sugar levels. They are slightly expensive and aren't really necessary. However, if you are serious about implementing this change, it is definitely a worthwhile investment.

Don't depend on this sort of behavior for too long. You need to learn all you need to know and move on. If eating becomes a big chore, it would be very hard to implement. At the beginning of it, it may be difficult.

Eating should be a natural response to hunger and it is perhaps something which is the hardest to learn. We often connect food to our emotions and social situations. Our brains would find it hard to disconnect these bonds.

If you find it tough to follow the recommendations according to the Glycemic Index, the best way is to focus all your energy on dealing with the emotions that you encounter when trying to break certain habits.

Our emotions are the reason why we sabotage our actions. Get books or watch videos that would help you deal better with the emotions that arise when you are trying to make this dietary change.

There are numerous good websites, books or support groups that help you overcome those emotional issues. It should be clear that no matter how hard it seems to live a healthy life, it would be even more difficult to make food changes when you need to cure yourself from any sort of illness. Prevention is better than cure, without a doubt.

The best thing to make this lifestyle change is to start now and slowly learn how to control your Glycemic Index. From here, pass these recommendations to your family. It is a great thing if children can start this habit while you are young as you would instill them for a lifetime of good health. As your children get older, they would be healthy unlike other people around them. They wouldn't struggle from diseases like diabetes or weight gain.

It is clear that it is very important that you follow the Glycemic Index and the bad effects of an overload of glucose. From here, you also learn what insulin is and the function is performs. Besides, you also read about the threat of diabetes and how complicated this disease could be. We also covered how eating right can prevent heart disease.

The great news is that with this information, you understand how the Glycemic Index diet works. The best benefits are that you have a healthy body, not just on the outside but on the inside as well. As you learn all about this, it is natural that you want to improve your health and assist your body to function better and more natural. It takes a bit of effort at the beginning but once you have mastered it, it would be truly effortless. Good luck!

Resource - Gluten Free Recipe Book

Fun With Gluten-Free, Low-Glycemic Food Cookbook is an ebook cookbook by Debbie Johnson, former owner and executive chef of The Golden Chalice Restaurant & Gallery, a 100% gluten-free, sugar-free, low-glycemic, organic, allergy-friendly establishment.

This is the first Cook-Book of its kind!

Every Recipe is Completely Gluten-Free, Sugar-Free (except fruit), Digestion-Friendly, Allergy-Friendly and Low Glycemic with Meat, Poultry, Fish meals and Tree-Nut-Free, Dairy-Free, Vegan and Vegetarian Options for most recipes.

Check it out at:

http://gluttenfreerecipes.wellbeingvalley.com/